HAPPY BABY

HAPPY SKIN

Expert Tips on Caring for Your Baby's Sensitive Skin

Allyson Peters

TABLE OF CONTENT

INTRODUCTION

Infant healthy skin is a fragile matter. In the early months, as your child's safe framework creates, you'll need to utilize the mildest cleaning agents and the littlest piece of moisturizer. Be that as it may, when dry diaper rash show up, now is the right time to treat those issues. When to start using those products should be discussed with your pediatrician. Your infant needs color free, aroma free child skin health management items. When you go shopping, be sure to carefully read the labels if you have a baby in your family. Child skin health management items that contain colors, scents, and synthetic substances can bother a child's skin and relaxing. Normal child skin health management items are alright for most babies. However, if you or someone in your family has asthma or allergies, your newborn may also be sensitive to some products' botanicals and herbs.

Hyperallergenic can be misleading. The term refers to the product's lower risk of triggering an allergic reaction; however, this does not necessarily imply that the product is more gentle on the skin than other products. Search for items that are phthalate-and without paraben. Babies may be affected by these chemicals.

Always keep in mind that your baby's skin deserves the best care, and following a proper skincare routine is important for their nutrition and overall health.

CHAPTER ONE

UNDERSTANDING BABY SKIN

Not at all like the skin of grown-ups, the skin of our little ones is as yet developing. Child's skin type could shift significantly, making it pretty much inclined to dermatitis, diaper rashes, awareness, and so on... The child's skin is sensitive, and the child's skin rashes are inclined to occur whenever. Realizing your child's skin type is the way to understanding what you can do when the rashes occur. You can handle it better the more you know.

All ethnic babies share one of five primary skin types: Dry, Normal Dry, Normal Sensitive, or Sensitive. Various kinds of skin rashes are connected with those five skin types. However, the newborn rash can occur on any type of skin and can be bothersome for both the baby and the parents.

SORTS OF CHILD SKIN

- *Dry Skin:*
  Abraded skin, flaky skin, scalp scratches, or, much more dreadful, irritated dermatitis could end up drying skin infants. The newborn's flaky skin may develop cracks, redness, and seborrheic dermatitis in some cases.

- *Ordinary Dry Skin and Typical Skin:*
  Some normal rash could happen to ordinary dry skin and typical skin, yet don't bother being stressed. Ensure the infant dry skin stays saturated.

There's a typical condition called milia. Milia are small, white, little knocks that seem to be pimples on an endearing face's. Those minuscule white knocks don't hurt. This skin issue for the most part vanishes inside a couple of days or weeks and needs no treatment.

- *Ordinary Touchy Skin:*

Ordinary touchy skin is the sort of skin condition that you might know about. On occasion, you may observe a few red spots on the baby's skin. Try not to stress excessively. A bug chomp or hypersensitive response may admirable motivation those red spots. It is entirely expected that a child's skin has an unfavorably susceptible response to specific materials or temperatures. Diaper rash, nappy rash, and intensity rash are exceptionally normal. Assuming a few little red knocks occur around the child's diaper region, the child may be delicate to the diaper changing item you use.

- *Delicate Skin:*

You need to give additional consideration to the delicate skin type. Skin rashes that occur on those touchy skins are more regrettable. Make sure to change the wet diaper straightaway to stay away from aggravation and intensity rash. Simply make sure to pick the regular diaper rash creams for your friends and family cautiously. Assuming the skin rash is getting extreme, if it's not too much trouble, counsel the specialist.

DIFFERENCES FROM ADULT SKIN

Baby skin is as yet creating in the initial not many long stretches of life. The skin is more slender, more delicate and more touchy. It is likewise less impervious to microorganisms, aggravations and allergens that might enter the skin and cause bothering. Newborn children have more slender skin than grown-ups. The papillae and veins enter further into the upper layer of the skin. The cells of your child's skin are more modest and put more extensive separated. This makes the skin more permeable.

Their epidermis is more slender and under-keratinized, contrasted and grown-ups. Accordingly, kids are in danger for expanded retention of specialists that can be retained through the skin.

Child skin isn't completely evolved until the kid is a half year old. Particularly the water-repellent horny layer is still exceptionally slender and the skin in this way loses much more water. Additionally, the number of additional skin cells is still lower than that of adults and children.

This makes it simple for microbes and general substances applied to the skin to enter child's sensitive skin. Babies must also be adequately shielded from UV rays due to the lack of fully developed melanin. . Sun protection that is appropriate for the child's age also becomes increasingly important to protect the child's delicate skin from long-term UV damage while playing and bathing.

Kids foster the skin construction and thickness of a grown-up from around one to two years old. However, because the body's surface area to weight ratio remains significantly higher, it is especially important to keep your baby's skin moist to prevent it from drying out.

BABY SKIN CONDITIONS

Skin conditions in babies and children might incorporate rashes, hives, moles, skin break out, pigmentations and that's just the beginning. These circumstances might be brought about by dermatitis, viral contaminations, bacterial contaminations, contagious diseases or different infections. Depending on the condition, treatments range from anti-itch creams to pain relievers and antibiotics. Different skin conditions can influence infants, babies, kids and teenagers all through their lives.

Conditions of the skin are not simply a cosmetic problem. The skin is the biggest organ of the body, and its capabilities are vital to the soundness of the other organ systems,The skin is a significant hindrance that forestalls over the top body liquid and mineral misfortune. It safeguards against contaminations and forestalls assimilation of harmful substances. It additionally manages body heat.

Child skin conditions can be brought about by different factors like intensity, cold, growth, microorganisms, slobbering, sensitivities or delayed contact with a wet nappy. Fortunately, the majority of skin conditions affecting infants are brief and self-limiting. In additional serious cases, notwithstanding, creams and balms, skin steroids, and oral prescription might be expected to determine the issue.

COMMON SKIN CONDITIONS IN BABIES

- **Heat rash:**

Which is also known as prickly heat or miliaria, is a type of rash that occurs in newborns due to the easily blocked sweat glands of their not-yet-developed sweat glands. It is especially common in humid, hot places like Singapore.

Rather than vanishing, sweat stays caught underneath the skin, causing aggravation and rash.

Symptoms:

Little, red to clear, pin-pointed knocks, generally over covered destinations like the back and rear end.

Causes:

Exorbitant sweat because of sweltering climate

Dressing a child too heartily or thick wrapping up

Dressing child in textures that don't permit sweat to ordinarily dissipate

- **Nappy rash**

Nappy rash, otherwise called diaper dermatitis, influences 35% of children eventually in their most memorable year of life. Its frequency tops at around 9 a year old enough.

Symptoms: A red, textured rash over the region of the skin that are covered by diapers.

Causes:

Delayed contact with pee and stools

Unreasonable dampness from delayed utilization of diapers

Grating from texture or glue tapes

Secondary disease from microbes or growth/yeast

- **Cradle cap:**

also known as seborrheic dermatitis, is a secondary infection caused by bacteria or fungus or yeast that typically manifests within the first few weeks of life and can persist for up to 4-6 months. Excessive moisture from prolonged diaper use Friction from fabric or adhesive tape

Support cap happens because of an excess of a typical skin parasite/yeast, optional to excitement from maternal chemicals while the child is still in the belly.

Be that as it may, in certain children, it very well might be an early indication of atopic dermatitis or atopic dermatitis.

Symptoms:

Layered, pink to red patches on the scalp. Some of the time, different region of the body are additionally impacted, for example the neck, armpits and crotch. Regions can give oily skin covered with flaky white or yellow scales.

Causes:An unusual creation of oil in the oil organs and hair follicles

Yeast/bacterial contamination

Atopic dermatitis

- **Atopic dermatitis,:**

otherwise called atopic dermatitis, is the most well-known skin condition influencing grown-ups and kids, including children. It influences up to 20 percent of school-matured kids in Singapore and for most patients, side effects start during the main year of life.

"Most kids with skin inflammation improve as they progress in years. In any case, the condition can repeat after months or even years. With great control, numerous patients with dermatitis can have solid, dynamic existences.

Symptoms:

Red, itchy, rough, and dry patches usually appear on a baby's cheeks and around the joints of their arms and legs.

Causes:

The specific reason for atopic dermatitis is obscure. Atopic eczema is an immune reaction that has been found to run in families and has a genetic component. Contributory elements which can go about as triggers or deteriorate the condition include:

Ecological factors, for example, high temperatures, house dust bugs, viral contaminations, immunizationsAllergens like cleansers, creams, cleansers

- **Getting teeth rash**

At the point when your child's teeth are beginning to come in, they might slobber much more than expected. Slobber can aggravate your child's skin. A harmless rash known as a teething rash can result from this. The rash causes little, red raised knocks on your endearing face's, neck or chest. Teething rashes may go away when your baby gets new teeth or stops drooling as much.

Getting teeth rashes don't cause fevers, so on the off chance that your child has a fever with a rash, talk with their medical care supplier. You can treat your child's getting teeth rash by keeping the region spotless and dry. You can likewise apply emollient cream to the impacted region. This might keep your child's slobber from bothering their skin.

CHAPTER TWO

ADVICE ON MAINTAINING HEALTHY INFANT SKIN

The behaviors of parents themselves might irritate their baby's skin; everything from burning aromatic candles in the room to leaving perfume or cologne on their skin and clothing to smoking habits can all potentially irritate a baby's skin or cause an allergic reaction. Even when parents are doing everything right for their child, their actions with regard to their bodies and skin nonetheless have an impact on that child's health.

A baby's skin is not only soft and seductive to pinch and snuggle, but it also acts as armor, thus skincare should reinforce that armor on your child.

SIMPLE WAYS TO CARE FOR YOUR BABY SKIN

Washing recurrence and procedure:

It depends on you how frequently you wash your child. While dermatologists' ideas shift from two or multiple times every week to washing everyday, they agree that the huge thing to do whatever it takes not to is dry out your youngster's skin.

You can work in a washing schedule consistently before sleep time, which can be alright for however long guardians are adding a moisturization normal too. (Keep in mind, the American Foundation of Pediatrics (AAP) suggests just giving your infant wipe showers until the umbilical line comes tumbles off. From that point onward, you can place your child in the water.)

Guardians can place themselves in a good position by tracking down the right size tub for their child and having every one of the items and washing frill inside arm's compass, so the child isn't left unattended, and furthermore filling the tub with around two creeps of tepid water to keep away from openness to outrageous water temperatures.

Utilizing a child washcloth, delicately purify the regions that should be scrubbed, like the diaper region, the folds of skin (armpits), and the feet.

"Truly, the remainder of the skin doesn't require cleanser each and every day, adding that a few times each seven day stretch of full-body purifying will get the job done. Furthermore, the explanation is on the grounds that children, as a general rule, lose a ton of dampness from their skin.

Shower time ought to simply last five to seven minutes, even on full-body purging days.

Wrap your baby immediately in a towel, preferably one with a hood, following a bath because babies' scalps can also lose a lot of heat.

In the wake of wiping your child off, promptly saturate to assist with fixing in hydration and safeguard their skin hindrance.

Saturating methods:

A child's skin is clinically dry in any event, when it doesn't show up so. Therefore, it is basic to apply a cream regardless of whether clear indications of dryness are not noticeable. After giving your baby a bath, it is very important to keep the water's moisture in so that the skin does not dry out and the skin barrier is refilled. Begin by wiping your child off (don't rub!), then, at that point, applying an emollient-style lotion in a meager layer all around their body. (Try not to let the cream develop in skin folds.) Furthermore, you can integrate saturating into your schedule a few times each day — perhaps as a decent back rub before rests or after a taking care of — particularly in the event that your child's skin feels or looks dry. What's more, foam it on yourself in the meantime!

You can apply cream, for example, Coconut Oil,Aloe Vera Gel, Shea Margarine.

Every day, give your baby an oil massage.

REALITIES ABOUT SATURATING:

In spite of the fact that oil knead has a few advantages, remembering further developing blood course for the child, the skin benefits rely upon the kind of oil utilized. It is likewise fundamental to saturate the child's skin following washing while it is as yet soggy to secure in the decency of the lotion and hydrate the skin.

In opposition to well known social ideas, the utilization of oils, particularly olive and mustard oil, are not great for rubs. These oils ought not be viewed alternative for lotions for infants. They might cause bothering, rashes and hypersensitive responses. All things considered, guardians ought to pick reasonable lotions that hydrate the child's skin.

In order to safeguard the baby's skin from dryness and other skin issues, it is essential to stress the significance of maintaining a moisturizing routine throughout the entire year. Creams are a non-oily moisturisation choice and are promptly consumed by the skin. Consequently, they are the most appropriate for use throughout the mid year months. Then again, child creams assist with giving the skin with a boundary that gives ultra-hydration and are the most ideal for dry to dry skin unnecessarily. They are suggested during cold and brutal winters when infants are more inclined to skin issues, including redness, dryness, white pieces, irritation, and stinging.

Appropriate diaper evolving:

Prior to starting, ensure all that you really want is helpful. Here is an agenda:

Change of garments for your child (if there should be an occurrence of a victory)

Changing table or evolving cushion/floor/bed/love seat

Diapers (material or dispensable)

Diaper cover or pins for material diapers, if necessary

Diaper cream or treatment

Dispensable pack

Wipes, delicate material, or cotton balls

Many individuals use child wipes to clean the diaper region. In any case, an infant's skin is very touchy. Utilizing warm water and a material or cotton balls during the initial not many long stretches of life can assist with forestalling skin bothering.

Purchasing wipes that are pre-saturated with water is another choice. Customary child wipes, particularly those containing liquor, can cause rashes and aggravation until youngsters are around 2 months old.

Bit by bit for how to change a diaper

- *Prepare*: To begin with, clean up. Then, at that point, accumulate your provisions. So that you don't have to turn your back while your baby is on the changing table, make sure you have everything you need within arm's reach but away from your baby.

- *Remove the Filthy Diaper*: Delicately lay your child on their back on the evolving surface. Loosen the diaper tabs or pins on each side. Then bring up your youngster's base off of the diaper by tenderly getting a handle on their lower legs and lifting them somewhat. On the off chance that there is a ton of stool in the diaper, you can utilize the upper portion of the diaper to clear it toward the lower half tenderly. Slide the diaper away. Keep it away from your baby but close by.
- *Clean Your Child's Skin*: Clean your child off. Utilize moistened cotton balls or wipes to thoroughly but gently clean the diaper area. While cleaning a vulva, consistently go from front to back to forestall disease. Keep in mind that you are only cleaning the vulva's exterior to get rid of any poop. Essentially, make certain to purge overall around a penis and scrotum completely. Furthermore, to try not to get peed on, place a spotless diaper or fabric over the penis while cleaning the diaper region. Put away the rubbish. Put any pre-owned expendable cleaning supplies on top of the dirty diaper.
- *Put on the Perfect Diaper*

Slide a perfect diaper under your child's base. Ensure the tabs are as an afterthought situated under your youngster's base. Colorful characters or markings mark the front of the majority of diapers today.

Prior to shutting the diaper, make certain to point a penis descending to forestall peeing out of the diaper. Apply any balms or creams you decide to utilize either as rash anticipation or treatment. Doing this step after you've put the new diaper under your child will assist with keeping you from being required to wipe balms off the evolving surface.

Even though baby powder was once a staple for changing diapers, experts like the American Academy of Pediatrics (AAP) do not recommend using it due to the health risks of inhaling airborne particles.

Then, close the new diaper. Pull the front between your youngster's legs and up over their stomach. Pull the diaper tabs open and around to the front, it is cozy however not excessively close to ensure the diaper. With material diapers, utilize the joined snaps or cautiously pin the diaper shut. To prevent irritation of the umbilical stump until it falls off, fold the front of the diaper down if you are not using specially cut newborn diapers.

- *Finish Up:*

While you clean, place your infant in a secure location, such as their crib or a baby carrier. Solidly roll up the filthy diaper and fold the tabs as far as possible over it. Place the diaper in a pack, diaper receptacle, or trash bin.

With material diapers, drop any crap into the latrine and flush away any remaining crap. Then, at that point, put the diaper into a container for the clothing.

Clean the evolving surface. Utilize a sanitizer to forestall tainting the following time you utilize the evolving table. At long last, clean up.

Clothing Decisions

Size 000 is expected to fit infants from 0-3 months, and size 00 is for children from 3-6 months. Some larger newborns may be ready to change into a size 00 right away. You could need to move up the sleeves, yet it will not be for a really long time.

Sizes change between kinds of garments and makers, so it merits contrasting garments with different pieces of clothing you as of now have, as opposed to depending just on the size on the mark.

Because babies grow so quickly, it's best to buy as few clothes as possible in each size.

Garments ought to be agreeable, delicate and simple to deal with.

Stretchy jumpsuits that secure at the front are ideal, as well as tops with envelope necks, which are simpler to move past your child's head. Jumpsuits with zips can make dressing your child speedy and simple as well.

Garments produced using cotton are a decent decision. In hot weather, cotton clothing will keep your child cooler than synthetic clothing. Cotton likewise washes well and is delicate against your child's touchy skin.

It means quite a bit to pay special attention to garments with a low fire risk mark. This label ought to be on jumpsuits and rompers for newborns.

Abstaining from purchasing infant garments with beading, strings, ties, drawstrings and attachments is ideal. These can be gagging dangers and strangulation or suffocation gambles.

Sun Security:

Your little one is sensitive in such countless ways, including that scrumptiously delicate, impeccable skin. Offspring of any age need to take care against the sun, however coddles under a half year face a one-two punch of not having the option to involve sunscreen and furthermore not having defensive melanins in their skin. In a dermatologist's ideal world, children's super-delicate skin wouldn't have any openness to that extraordinary chunk of fire, however except if you anticipate living in a dull cavern, your novice is probably going to get a couple of beams.

A few pointers to protect your baby's epidermis are as follows:

Stay inside during the day, add some shade, cover up, limit exposure to the sun, set up a tent if you're on the beach, apply sunscreen at six months, wear a hat, and cover your car seat and   stroller.

CHAPTER THREE

PRODUCTS FOR BABY SKIN CARE

Infant healthy skin is a sensitive matter. In the early months, as your child's safe framework creates, you'll need to utilize the mildest chemicals and the littlest piece of moisturizer. Child healthy skin items that contain colors, scents, and synthetic compounds can bother a child's skin and relaxing. The majority of infants can use natural baby skin care products safely. The best way to protect baby's skin is to choose products that are both safe and effective. Newborn Skin Care Products As the nursery is set up, put together these products for baby's skin:

SOME NORMAL CHILD SKIN HEALTH MANAGEMENT ITEMS AND HOW TO UTILIZE THEM:

- *Baby Cleanser or Chemical*: Utilize a gentle and scent free child cleanser or cleaning agent to tenderly purge your child's skin during shower time. Wet your child's body with warm water, apply a modest quantity of cleanser or cleaning agent to a washcloth or your hands, and delicately knead it onto your child's skin. Pat dry after thoroughly rinsing with warm water.

- *Baby Cleanser:* Clean your baby's hair and scalp with a tear-free baby shampoo. Wet your child's hair with warm water, apply a limited
- quantity of cleanser, and delicately rub it into the hair and scalp. Flush completely with warm water.

- *Baby Moisturizer*: Apply a delicate and hypoallergenic child cream to saturate and safeguard your child's skin. After shower time or at whatever point your child's skin feels dry, take a modest quantity of salve and delicately knead it onto your child's skin until it is retained.

- *Baby Cream:* Utilize a diaper cream to forestall and treat diaper rash. Clean your child's base with warm water and a delicate wipe, wipe off, and afterward apply a flimsy layer of diaper cream to the impacted region. Try to apply it equitably and cover the whole diaper region.

- *Sunscreen*: In the event that your child is more established than a half year, apply a child safe sunscreen with SPF 30 or higher to shield their sensitive skin from the sun's destructive beams. Apply a liberal measure of sunscreen to all uncovered region of your child's skin something like 15 minutes prior to heading outside. Reapply like clockwork or in the wake of swimming or perspiring.

Make sure to constantly fix test new items prior to utilizing them on your child's whole body and talk with a pediatrician in the event that you have any worries or inquiries concerning explicit items or your child's skin health management schedule.

CHAPTER FOUR

CONCLUSION

Subsequent to directing exhaustive exploration and examination on the subject of Baby skin care management, obviously the main component to consider is the utilization of protected, delicate, and regular items. Cruel synthetic compounds and engineered fixings can make harm and bothering a child's sensitive skin.

Notwithstanding item choice, it is vital to lay out a reliable skincare routine for children to keep up with skin wellbeing and forestall any potential issues like dryness or rashes. This routine ought to incorporate ordinary showers, delicate purifying, and saturating.

Parents must also stay up to date on the most recent research and recommendations for baby skin care. Talking with a medical services proficient or expert can give important knowledge and direction.

Generally speaking, focusing on the utilization of protected and normal items, laying out a steady skincare schedule, and remaining informed on prescribed procedures are key variables in guaranteeing ideal child skin wellbeing and care.